ICS 11.020

SCM

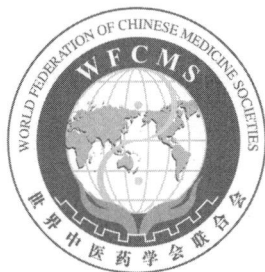

世界中医药学会联合会

World Federation of Chinese Medicine Societies

Standard of WFCMS   SCM 0026–2019

浮针疗法技术操作规范

Standardized Manipulations of Fu's Subcutaneous Needling

2019 年 3 月 29 日发布实施

中国健康传媒集团·北京
中国医药科技出版社

图书在版编目（CIP）数据

浮针疗法技术操作规范/世界中医药学会联合会组织编写. — 北京：中国医药科技出版社，2019.9
（2025. 6 重印）

ISBN 978-7-5214-1349-6

Ⅰ.①浮… Ⅱ.①世… Ⅲ.①针刺疗法—技术规范 Ⅳ.① R245.3-65

中国版本图书馆 CIP 数据核字（2019）第 205750 号

美术编辑 陈君杞
版式设计 南博文化

出版 **中国健康传媒集团** | 中国医药科技出版社
地址 北京市海淀区文慧园北路甲 22 号
邮编 100082
电话 发行：010-62227427 邮购：010-62236938
网址 www. cmstp. com
规格 880 × 1230mm $^1/_{16}$
印张 2 $^1/_2$
字数 56 千字
版次 2019 年 9 月第 1 版
印次 2025 年 6 月第 4 次印刷
印刷 三河市万龙印装有限公司
经销 全国各地新华书店
书号 ISBN 978-7-5214-1349-6
定价 **26.00 元**

获取新书信息、投稿、为图书纠错，请扫码联系我们。

目　　次

前　言

本《规范》的主要起草单位：世界中医药学会联合会浮针专业委员会。

本《规范》参与起草的单位：南京浮针医学研究所、广东省中医院。

本《规范》主要起草人：符仲华、孙健。

本《规范》参与起草人及审阅专家（按姓氏拼音排序）：

中国：郝晓明、李桂凤、王文涛。

英国：吴继东。

中国台湾：周立伟。

中国香港：袁康就。

中国澳门：卢得健。

伊朗：Amir Hooman Kazemi。

本《规范》的起草程序遵守了世界中医药学会联合会发布的SCM 0001-2009《标准制定和发布工作规范》。

本《规范》由世界中医药学会联合会发布，版权归世界中医药学会联合会所有。

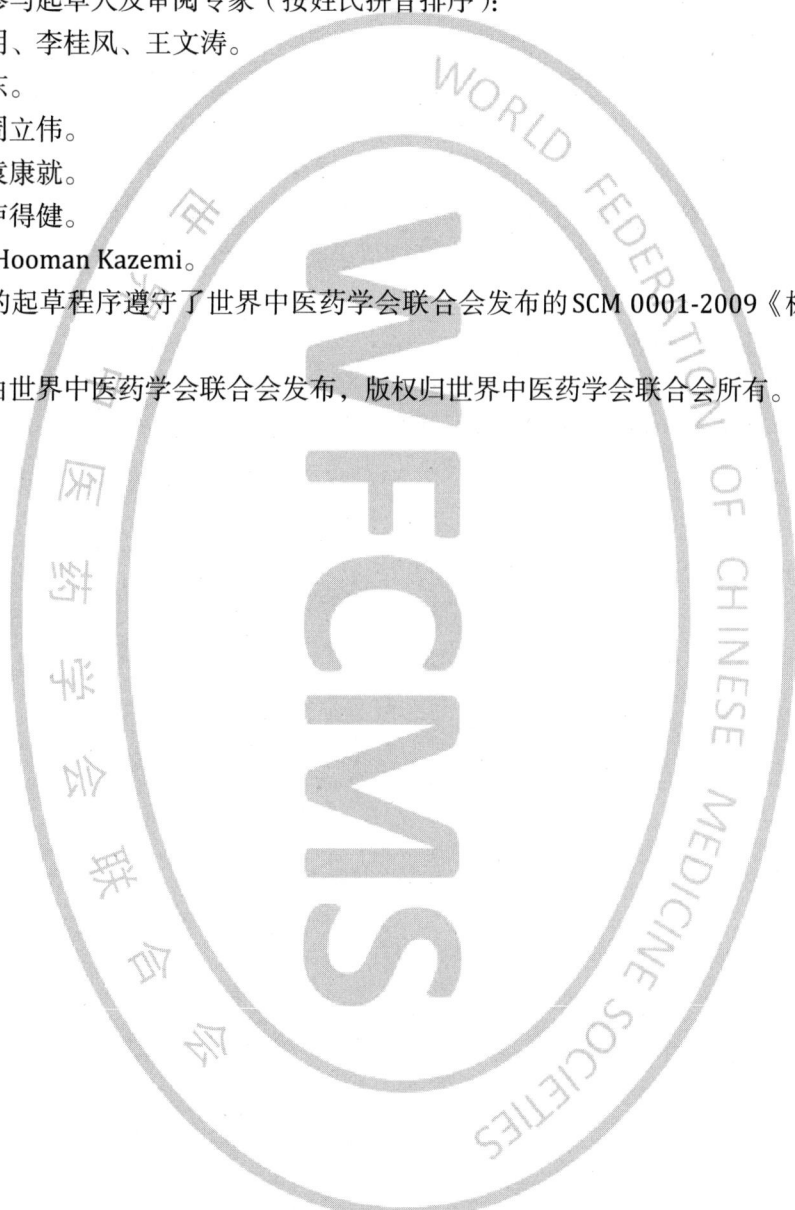

引　言

浮针疗法源于经典，基于临床，继承创新，是符仲华浮针医学团队历经20余年获得的科研成果，是具有自主知识产权的原始创新技术。浮针疗法安全、无毒副作用，患者容易接受。

为了方便临床学习和应用，加强浮针教学培训的标准化，使浮针临床操作规范化，特起草了《浮针疗法操作技术规范》，对浮针疗法的术语和定义、适应证与禁忌证、操作步骤、异常情况及处理、注意事项等方面进行规范化和标准化规定。

本文件的发布机构请注意，声明符合本文件时，可能涉及到一次性使用浮针与浮针进针器相关专利的使用。

本文件的发布机构对于该专利的真实性、有效性和范围无任何立场。

该专利持有人已向本文件的发布机构保证，他愿意同任何申请人在合理且无歧视的条款和条件下，就专利授权许可进行谈判，该专利持有人的声明已在本文件的发布机构备案。

相关信息可以通过以下联系方式获得：

专利持有人姓名：符仲华

地址：北京市大兴区世界之花假日广场D座738室

请注意本文件的某些内容可能涉及专利。本文件的发布机构不承担识别这些专利的责任。

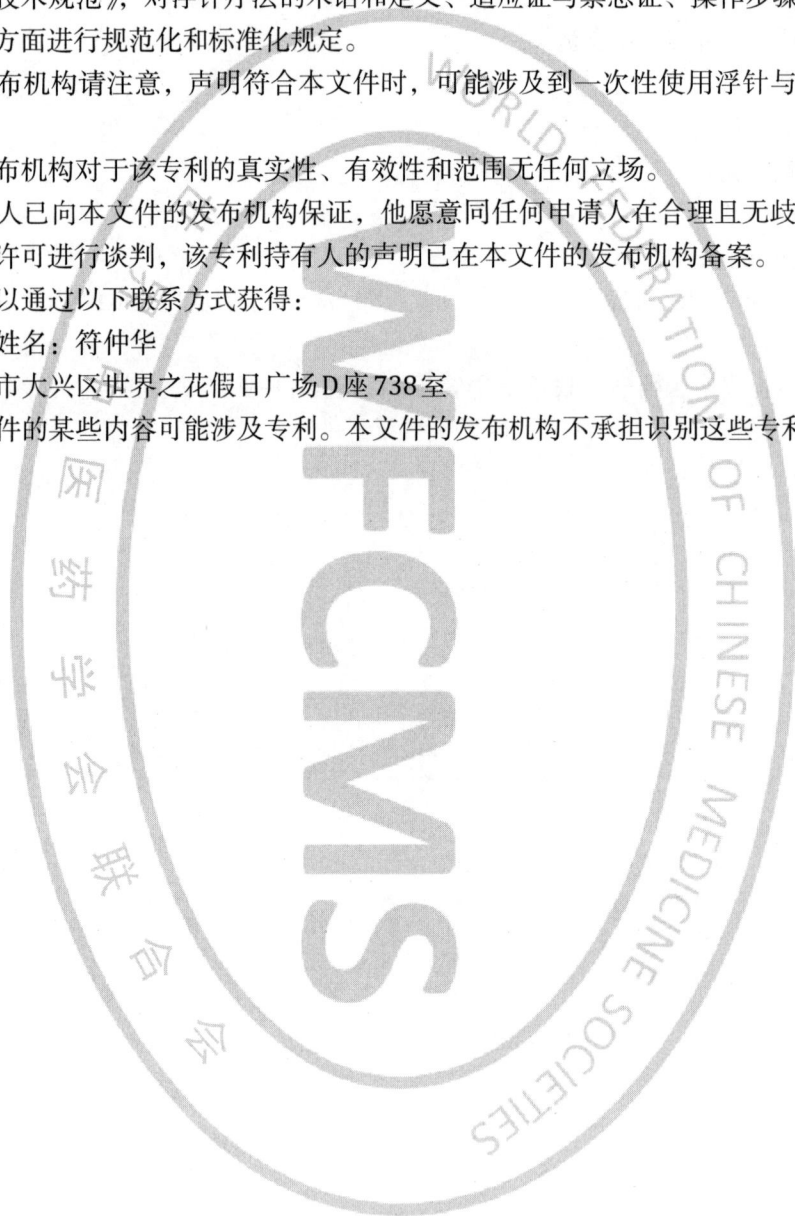

浮针疗法技术操作规范

1 范围

本《规范》规定了浮针疗法的术语和定义、适应证与禁忌证、操作步骤及要求、异常情况及处理、注意事项等。

本《规范》适用于浮针疗法技术的操作。

2 规范性引用文件

本《规范》无规范性引用文件。

3 术语和定义

下列术语和定义适用于本文件。

3.1

浮针疗法

用一次性使用浮针等针具，在引起局限性病痛的紧张性肌肉周围或邻近四肢进针，并进行扫散操作的皮下针刺法。

3.2

患肌

在运动中枢正常的情况下，放松状态时依旧紧张的肌肉。

3.3

肌肉前病痛

指可以导致肌肉慢性缺血缺氧，引起肌肉及其附属结构产生病理性紧张的病痛。

3.4

肌肉中病痛

由于慢性缺血缺氧、肌肉本身及其附属结构产生病理性紧张所引发的病痛。

3.5

肌肉后病痛

肌肉的病理性紧张影响到分布于肌肉内、肌肉周边，并与该肌肉紧密相关的其他器官（如动脉、静脉、神经等）而产生的一系列病痛。

3.6

运针

浮针刺入皮下后，沿皮下向前刺入适当深度的一段操作过程。

3.7

扫散

运针完毕后，将针身在皮下平行左右摆动的一系列动作。

3.8

再灌注活动

在短时间主动或被动大力收缩患肌，然后再放松的活动。经常在收缩患肌时，医务人员给予等力阻抗。多用在浮针操作过程中。对轻度不适，也有单独使用的情况。

4 适应证与禁忌证

4.1 适应证

4.1.1 肌肉前疾病

强直性脊柱炎、类风湿关节炎、哮喘、痛风、帕金森病、面瘫、肩关节周围炎等。

4.1.2 肌肉中疾病

颈椎病、网球肘、腰椎间盘突出症、慢性膝关节痛、踝关节扭伤、头痛、前列腺炎、漏尿、呃逆、失眠、抑郁、慢性咳嗽、习惯性便秘等。

4.1.3 肌肉后疾病

头昏、眩晕、心慌胸闷、局部麻木、局部水肿、乳腺增生、冷症、黄斑变性、糖尿病足、股骨头缺血性坏死、骨性变化等。

4.2 禁忌证

4.2.1 有传染病、恶性病的患者，或有急性炎症、发热的患者。

4.2.2 常有自发性出血或凝血功能障碍导致损伤后出血不止者。

4.2.3 皮肤有感染、溃疡、瘢痕或肿瘤的部位。

5 操作步骤及要求

5.1 进针点选择

临床依据以下原则确定进针点。

a）多数情况下，进针点选择在患肌周围、距离患肌 3 ～ 5cm 处，上、下、左、右或斜取皆可。

b）小范围、少患肌进针点宜近，大范围、多患肌进针点宜远。

c）从远到近。尤其是对于区域内多个患肌，如慢性颈腰部疼痛，多伴有上肢和下肢的异常，进针点的选取要从远到近，而不是相反。

5.2 针具选择及体位选择

5.2.1 针具选择

针灸临床所使用的浮针进针器和一次性使用浮针均应符合中国医疗器械生产和销售监督法规的规定（附录 A）。为防止针刺意外事故的发生，一次性使用浮针在每次使用前，均应严格检查，如发现包装损坏等不合格现象，予以剔除。

5.2.2 体位选择

在浮针操作时常用的体位如下。

a）仰卧位：主要适宜于取头、胸、腹部进针点和上下肢部位的进针点。

b）侧卧位：主要适宜于在身体侧面和上下肢部位的进针点和治疗。

c）俯卧位：主要适宜于在头、脊背、腰臀部和下肢背侧的进针点。胸下垫枕，双手交叉，置于前头部。

d）坐位：主要适宜于颈肩部、上背部、上肢、膝关节和下肢部位的进针点。

e）俯伏坐位：适宜于后枕部、上颈部进针点的操作。

5.3 消毒和进针

5.3.1 消毒

进针部位消毒：常规皮肤消毒。

进针器可以一次性使用，也可前端消毒：使用前，用酒精棉球擦拭消毒进针器前端。

5.3.2 进针

将去除保护套的一次性使用浮针突点面向上，放入进针器传动杆，向后拉入固定，中指托在进针器底座下，示指扣在红色按钮上，拇指置在进针器上面。（图1）

将进针器前端放置在消毒过的进针点的皮肤上，进针器与皮肤角度尽可能要小，左手配合，前推下压，按动按钮，将浮针快速刺入皮下层。（图2）

左手拇指和示指持浮针针座，从固定槽中上抬，右手将进针器向后退出。（图3）

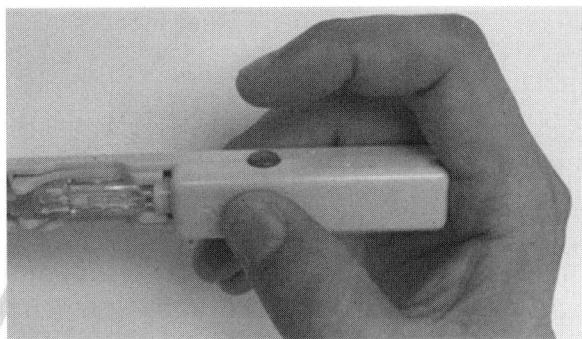

图1　握持进针器的姿势

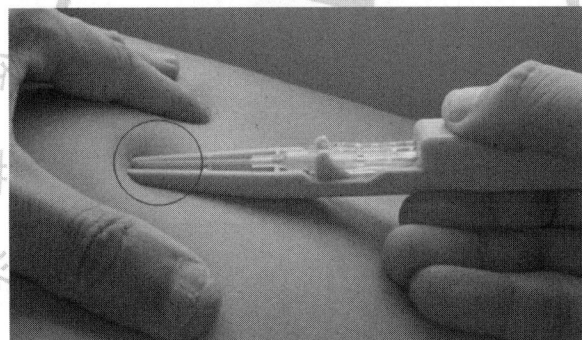

图2　进针前进针器与皮肤之间的关系

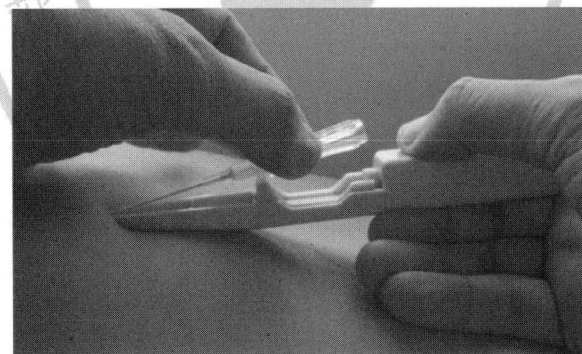

图3　进针后右手固定，左手提捏浮针

5.4　运针、扫散

5.4.1　运针

进针后，若浮针针尖直接进入了肌层，患者有酸胀感，医生持针的手指能够感觉到阻力，这时可用拇指、示指和中指提捏针柄，然后轻柔、缓慢向后提拉针身，使针尖离开肌层，退至皮下。

确保浮针针尖在皮下后，即可放倒针身，做好运针准备。运针时，单用右手持针，使针体沿皮下向前推进，推进时将针体稍稍提起，使针尖略微翘起，使针尖不深入肌层。运针时可见皮肤呈线状隆起。如果在运针过程中，患者突感刺痛，或者医生突感阻力，多半是因为针尖刺到血管壁。因此，运针过程能慢则慢，如医生突感阻力而患者还没有感觉到刺痛，迅速将针稍退，然后或向上或向下调整针尖方向，避免刺痛患者。

一般以软套管全部埋入皮下为度。部分情况下，如在手指关节侧面或者其他小关节附近进针，软套管不必全部埋入皮下。

5.4.2 扫散

5.4.2.1 扫散操作方法

运针到位后，左手固定软管座，右手退后针芯，将软管座上的突起固定于芯座上的卡槽内，这时，针芯的针尖已经退回软套管内，不再外露，而是几乎与软套管平齐。

扫散时，用右手拇指内侧指甲缘和中指夹持芯座，示指和无名指分居中指左右两边，拇指尖固定在皮肤上作为支点，示指和无名指一前一后作跷跷板样扇形扫散动作。扫散动作幅度宜大，平稳有力，节律宜慢，避免产生酸麻胀痛等感觉。扫散过程中，右手操作，左手配合再灌注活动。

5.4.2.2 扫散的种类

临床上根据针体摆动的方式不同，将扫散分为如下两类。

a）平扫：平扫是指针尖在同一水平面上左右摆动，平扫较为省力，比较常用，适合大多数情况。现在因为有了再灌注活动的配合，临床大多数选用平扫操作。

b）旋扫：针体沿着顺时针或者逆时针方向做椭圆运动，适用于比较顽固的病痛。（图4）

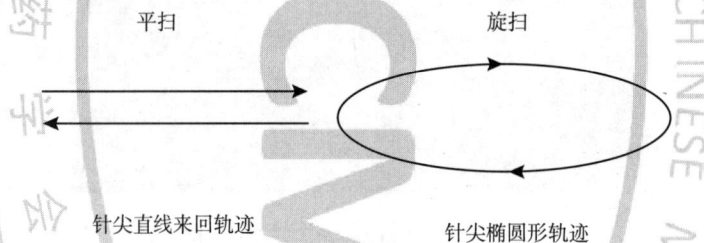

平扫   旋扫

针尖直线来回轨迹   针尖椭圆形轨迹

图4 平扫和旋扫

5.4.2.3 扫散的时间、频率

一个进针点的扫散时间约为2分钟，次数为200次左右，一般每扫散半分钟，即可检查、评估患肌的变化情况。评估后，发现已经缓解，即可停止扫散。

5.5 再灌注活动

5.5.1 再灌注活动的分类

5.5.1.1 主动再灌注活动

患者在没有辅助情况下主动完成的再灌注活动。

5.5.1.2 被动再灌注活动

患者不能自主完成，需要依靠外力帮助完成的再灌注活动。

5.5.2 再灌注活动的操作要求

5.5.2.1 幅度大

根据患肌的解剖功能活动，引导患者做到肌肉的最大幅度（等张收缩）或者最大强度（等长收缩）。

5.5.2.2 速度慢

最大幅度、最大强度和放松时都要有1～3秒停顿，完成一个再灌注活动建议在10秒左右。

5.5.2.3 次数少

每次连续的同样方向、同样角度的动作，即同一组再灌注活动动作，以不超过3次为宜。

5.5.2.4 间隔长

同一组患肌完成一组再灌注活动后，至少半小时内不要进行下一组再灌注活动，使肌肉得到充分休息、放松。

5.5.2.5 变化多

对于顽固性疼痛，可针对性改变再灌注活动。

5.5.3 再灌注活动的操作方法

临床操作时应结合与病痛相关的患肌肌肉的走向、关节特征，来设计再灌注活动；不同部位的再灌注活动有所不同。

 a）颈部：采用低头、抬头、左侧头、右侧头、左旋头、右旋头等六大动作。

 b）肩部：采用梳头、后背、上举等动作。

 c）腰部：采用抱头弓腰、大小飞燕、左右扭臀、原地踏步、自主咳嗽等动作。

 d）膝盖：采用屈伸、原地踏步等动作。

 e）胸部、背部：采用深呼吸、自主咳嗽等动作。

5.6 留管及取管

5.6.1 留管操作

扫散完毕，抽出针芯放回保护套管内，用纸质胶布（或胶质胶布）贴附于管座，将管座固定在皮肤上，胶布大小保证覆盖整个管座，以固定留于皮下的软套管。

5.6.2 留管时间

结合临床实际情况，一般建议留管1小时为宜。医生可根据天气情况、患者的反应和病情的性质决定留管时间的长短。天气炎热、易出汗或患者因胶布过敏等因素造成针口或局部皮肤瘙痒，时间不宜过长；反之则留管时间可适当延长。

5.6.3 取管

取管时一般以左手拇指、示指按住针孔周围皮肤，右手拇、示指两指捏住软管座，缓慢将软管取出，用消毒干棉球按压针孔，防止出血。取管后，患者休息片刻即可离开。

5.7 浮针治疗间隔时间和疗程

5.7.1 间隔时间

慢性病痛，一般每日治疗1次，连续治疗2～3天，此后可逐渐延长治疗间隔，2～3天做1次治疗；其余视疗效调整治疗方案。

5.7.2 疗程

一般以3次为1个疗程。

6 异常情况及处理

6.1 皮下瘀血

微量皮下出血及局部的小块青紫可自行消退，一般不必特殊处理，但需向患者做好解释工作，以消除患者顾虑情绪及恐惧心理。

若局部肿胀、疼痛明显，青紫面积较大而影响到功能活动时，需出针并冷敷止血，24小时后再热敷及局部轻轻按揉以促进瘀血消散。

6.2 晕针

6.2.1 预防晕针

做好解释、沟通工作，消除患者紧张情绪，选用合适体位，治疗时手法轻柔。若患者饥饿或疲劳，应嘱其进食、休息、饮水后再予针刺。过于紧张者，可以采用卧位进针。针刺治疗过程医生要注意观察患者神色，询问患者感觉，一旦有头晕、胸闷、心慌等晕针先兆，应立即停止治疗，及早采取处理措施。

6.2.2 晕针处理

立即停止针刺活动，出针，使患者平卧，注意保暖，轻者仰卧片刻，饮用适量温开水或糖水后，即可恢复正常。若仍有不省人事、呼吸微弱、血压下降者，可考虑配合其他治疗或采用急救措施。

7 注意事项

7.1 浮针治疗前应简要向患者解释浮针的操作和特点，消除患者对浮针的恐惧感和疑虑。

7.2 对于年老体弱、初次治疗、恐惧扎针者宜尽量采用卧位治疗。

7.3 再灌注活动时，活动范围需由小到大，循序渐进，外加负荷力量应由轻到重。主动再灌注活动时，负荷力量为反作用力；被动再灌注活动时，禁止突然发力或大力活动患者关节等。注意结合患者年龄、体质、精神状态等因素，因人制宜实施再灌注活动，避免一次再灌注活动时间过长、过于用力或者过于频繁。

7.4 留管期间保持局部清洁干燥，防止感染。留管期间可适当活动，但活动范围不宜过大，以免影响软套管的固定。少数情况下，若留置于皮下的软套管移动后触及血管，导致刺痛或出血，即可取出软管。留管局部有瘙痒感觉时，无需紧张，多为胶布过敏所致，医生可改用其他类型物件固定，如止血贴等。

7.5 妇女怀孕3个月以内者，不宜在小腹部针刺。若怀孕3个月以上者，腹部、腰骶部也不宜针刺。如果孕妇紧张，一定不要针刺。

7.6 在局部涂抹过红花油、按摩乳等刺激性外用药，或者用过强力膏药、强力火罐及刮痧的局部，在短时间内不宜浮针治疗；如果经以上外用药、膏药、火罐等治疗后，局部皮肤状态已经恢复正常，则适合用浮针疗法。

7.7 局部短期内接受过封闭疗法治疗者不宜用浮针治疗。

附录 A
（规范性附录）
浮针针具的结构和规格

A.1 进针器

浮针进针器作为浮针专用配套工具，由南京浮针医学研究所研发。应用该浮针进针器可以降低针刺时的痛苦，方便医生的进针操作，确保进针部位的准确和进针过程的安全。

进针器组成由四部分组成，分别是底座、控制按钮、进针器传动杆和固定槽。（图A.1）

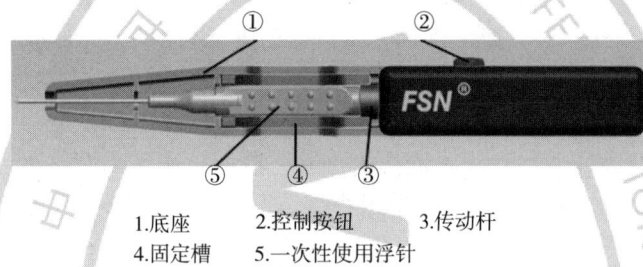

1.底座　2.控制按钮　3.传动杆
4.固定槽　5.一次性使用浮针

图 A.1　已安装浮针的进针器

A.2 浮针针具

A.2.1 浮针的结构

复式结构，分为三部分。浮针针具的三个组成部分的组合顺序见图A.2。

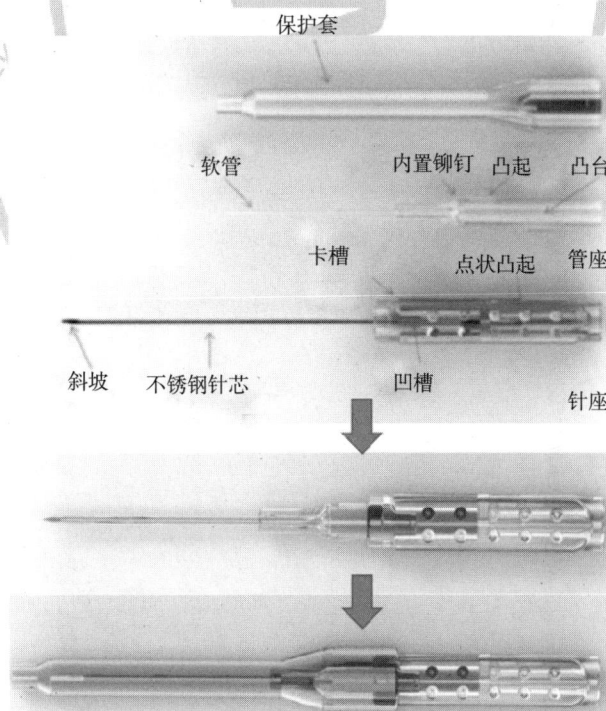

图 A.2　浮针结构和部件

A.2.1.1 针芯

针芯由不锈钢针和硬塑料的芯座组成（图A.2）。该部分使浮针达到足够的刚性以快速进入人体，并完成扫散动作。不锈钢针的针尖呈斜坡形。针芯座的其中一面分布有点状突起，当凸点向上时针尖斜面也向上。该面与针尖的斜坡一致，针芯座前端有一纵向凹槽，凹槽前段右侧有一横向卡槽，用于扫散时固定软套管。

A.2.1.2 软套管及管座

软套管内包不锈钢针（钢针在里，软套管在外），通过内置的铆钉固定在塑料管座上（图A.2）。管座上有一突起，与芯座上的凹槽及其卡槽相配套。平时管座上的突起置于凹槽底部，扫散时该突起当放置于卡槽内。

软套管的主要作用如下。

a）软管座和芯座吻合为一体，有利于进针、运针和扫散时的稳定。

b）扫散时不锈钢针针尖完全退入软套管，可避免针尖伤及血管等组织引起刺痛。

c）因其具有足够的柔软度，治疗结束后可以留置于皮下数小时，不会刺伤血管和其他组织，不影响正常活动。

A.2.1.3 保护套管

为保护不锈钢针和软套管不与它物碰撞产生磨损，同时也为了有利于保持无菌状态，浮针采用了保护套管（图A.2）。扫散完毕后，针芯不能随意丢弃，必须重新放回保护套管内，以防止刺伤自己和他人。

A.2.2 浮针的长度、直径、外观及保存

A.2.2.1 浮针外观

浮针全称为一次性使用浮针，又称为一次性使用皮下套管针灸针（图A.3）。现在使用的浮针规格，见表A.1。

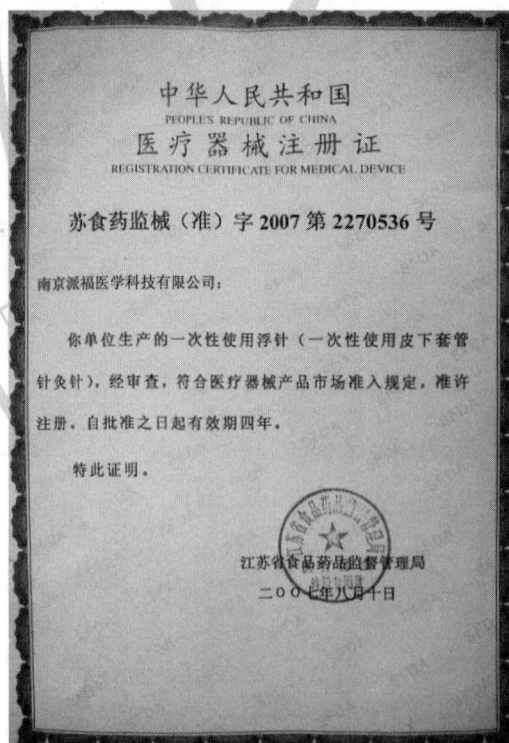

图A.3 一次性使用浮针又称为一次性使用皮下套管针灸针

浮针针具只运用一种型号，即当初发明初期计划的中号。

表 A.1　浮针针芯的规格尺寸

	枕芯（mm）	软套管（mm）
长度	52	49
直径	0.6	1.05（外径）

A.2.2.2　浮针的使用和保存

浮针针具是无菌产品，供一次性使用，包装破损后请勿使用。打开包装后，检查浮针表面是否光洁、有无毛糙及加工缺陷，软管是否透明，浮针针尖是否锋利、有无毛刺和弯钩等缺陷，若发现上述问题，请停止使用，并通报生产厂家，由厂家处理。

浮针针具请保存在干燥、无热源的地方。

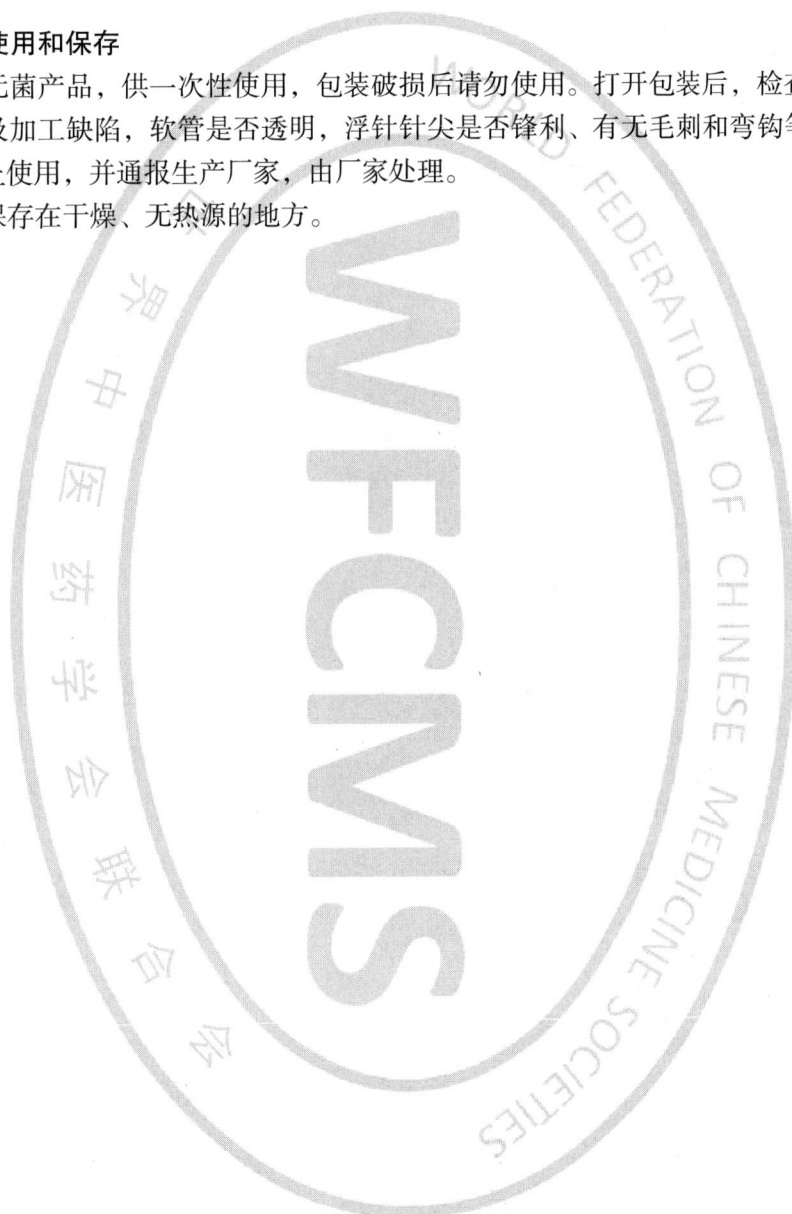

附录 B
（资料性附录）
患肌的特征、分级、临床表现及检查方法

B.1 患肌的基本特征与临床分级

B.1.1 基本特征

运动中枢正常的患者在被检查区域放松的情况下，医生用指腹触摸目标肌肉时，有"紧、僵、硬、滑"的感觉，患者局部常有酸胀不适、疼痛，或者有明显异常感，与患肌相关的关节常有乏力感。相关关节活动范围常常减小。

B.1.2 临床分级

临床中把肌肉的紧张状态分为5个等级，具体界定如下。

-：肌肉柔软，活动正常。

+：肌肉轻度紧张，没有明显临床症状。

++：肌肉明显紧张、僵硬，多伴有轻度的疼痛等症状，休息后常可缓解。

+++：肌肉中度紧张、僵硬，伴随相关部位的疼痛等症状。

++++：肌肉重度紧张、僵硬，肌腹可触及滑动团块或条索样改变，伴随严重的不能忍受的疼痛等症状，休息后缓解不明显，甚至影响正常生活。

B.2 患肌的临床表现

患肌的临床表现主要有五大类，分别为患肌直接引起、患肌间接引起、由肌性内脏引起的病症，以及部分情绪睡眠障碍和部分不明原因的病症。

B.2.1 第一大类

患肌直接引起的临床主诉：疼痛、功能障碍、乏力。主要病症包括：颈椎病、网球肘、腰椎间盘突出症、慢性膝关节痛、踝关节扭伤等。

肌肉引发的疼痛的特征如下。

a）疼痛性质多为酸痛、胀痛，少有刺痛。

b）定位往往不准确，只能指出大概方位。

c）经常会影响到周边肌肉组织或者协同肌。

d）这种疼痛大部分喜热敷、喜按摩，不喜压力，如果仅仅触碰或者摩擦皮肤，对这种疼痛没有影响。

e）遇天气转凉、相关肌肉劳累、睡眠不足、情绪不佳时这种疼痛往往加重。

f）使用非甾体类镇痛药后、相关肌肉得到休息后、天气转暖后、按摩后、情绪愉悦时疼痛往往减轻。

g）长久的疼痛常常引发相关骨骼、关节的变化，如骨质增生、假性滑脱、脊柱侧弯、膝关节变形等。

B.2.2 第二大类

患肌影响其内部或邻近的神经、动脉、静脉引起。

a）神经相关：主要表现为患肌下游病症，如麻木感。

b）动脉相关：表现为患肌的相关病症，如头痛、眩晕、畏寒、怕冷、触温下降，甚至整个肢体冰冷感。

c）静脉相关：表现为患肌下游病症，如水肿、酸胀、瘙痒、肤色变暗等。

B.2.3　第三大类

邻近骨骼肌的病理性紧张与肌性内脏的病变同时发作，二者之间有很密切的联系，两者常常同时出现，治疗后同时消失。

人体不同系统的患肌临床表现如下。

a）呼吸系统平滑肌：干咳、久咳、哮喘、胸闷气促、呼吸不畅等。

b）心肌：胸闷、心慌、气短、胸痛等。

c）胃肠平滑肌：胃痛胃胀、烧心反酸、嗳气欲呕、食欲不振、消瘦、习惯性便秘、慢性腹泻、畏惧凉食冷饮等。

d）泌尿系统平滑肌：尿频、尿急、尿不尽、尿无力、输尿管结石、漏尿等。

e）生殖泌尿系统平滑肌：

女性：痛经、月经异常、经行不畅等。

男性：阳痿不举等。

B.2.4　第四大类

情绪和睡眠相关病症如焦虑、失眠、情绪波动大。

B.2.5　第五大类

不明原因的一类病症，出现自主神经机能失调的症状以及本体感受性失调。

自主神经机能失调的症状，如异常的出汗、持续的流泪、持续的卡他性鼻炎、过度的流涎、心前区不适、竖毛活动；本体感受性失调，如不平衡、眩晕、耳鸣，还有举起无力、重量感知紊乱。

B.3　患肌的检查方法

a）标记出患者告知的病痛处。

b）根据解剖和生物力学知识罗列所有可能为患肌的肌肉。

c）用拇指指腹或示指、中指、无名指三个手指指腹并在一起，触摸怀疑为患肌的肌腹的紧张度，紧张度较周围肌增高时，确定为患肌。

SCM 0026-2019

参考文献

［1］ 符仲华.浮针医学纲要［M］.北京：人民卫生出版社，2016.
［2］ 符仲华.浮针疗法治疗疼痛手册［M］.北京：人民卫生出版社，2011.

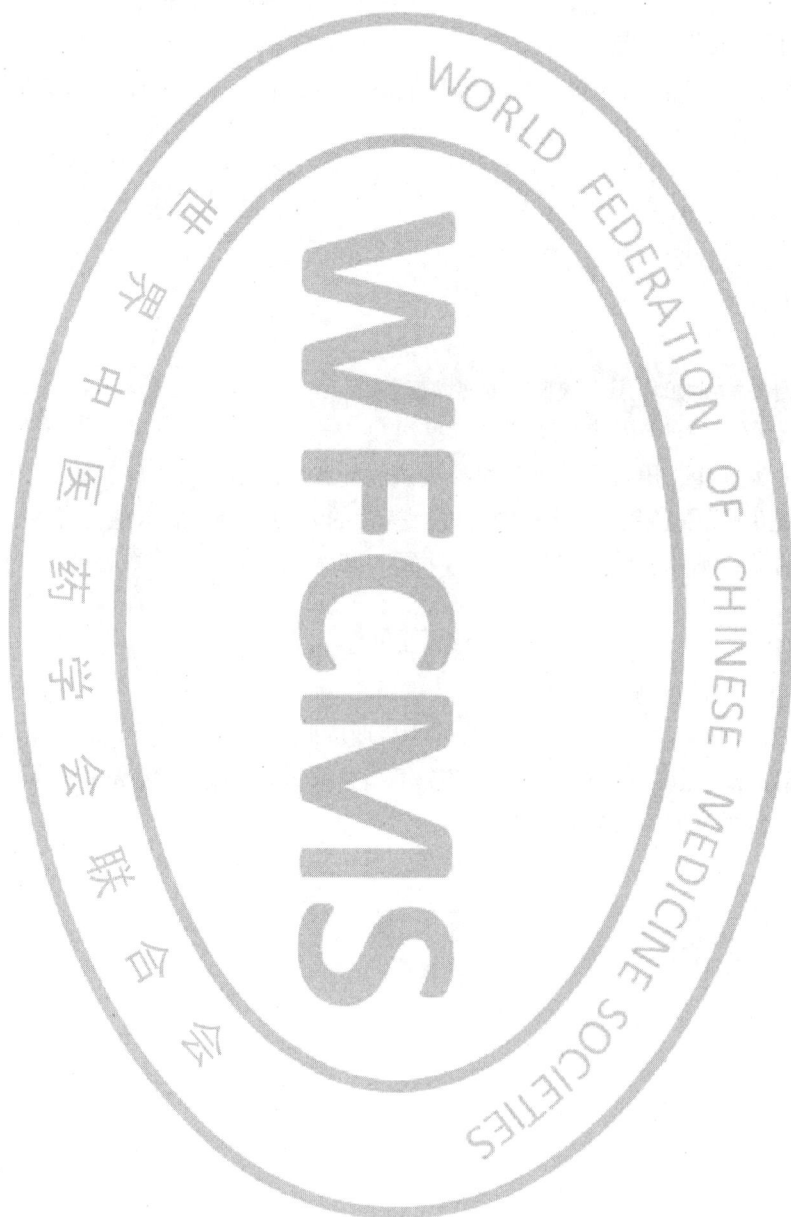

Foreword

The drafting designer: Specialty Committee of Fu's Subcutaneous Needling of World Federation of Chinese Medicine Societies.

Other participating institutions for the standard: Nanjing FSN Medical Institute, Guangdong Provincial Hospital of TCM.

The chief contributors of this standard: Fu Zhonghua, Sun Jian.

Other participants and review experts are (sorted by surname phonetic alphabet):

China: Hao Xiaoming, Li Guifeng, Wang Wentao.

UK: Wu Jidong.

China Taiwan: Chou Liwei.

China HongKong: Yuan Kangjiu.

China Macau: Lu Dejian.

Iran: Amir Hooman Kazemi.

This standard complies with SCM 0001-2009 *Specification for making and release of Standard and its Publication* released by World Federation of Chinese Medicine Societies.

This standard is issued by the Federation of World Chinese Medicine Societies and its copyright belongs to the World Federation of Chinese Medicine Societies.

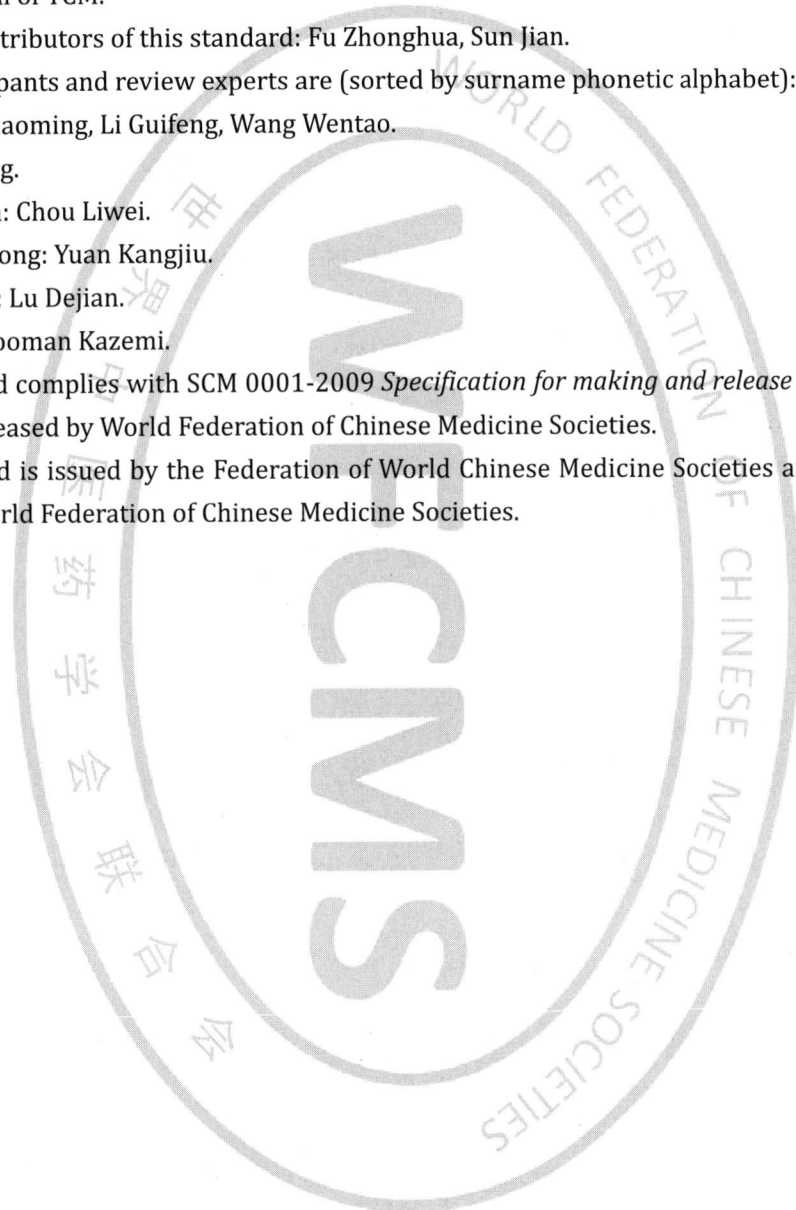

Introduction

Fu's Subcutaneous Needling (FSN) therapy is originated from classics and based on clinical practice. Out of inheritance and innovation, it is the scientific research achievement of Fu Zhonghua and his research team over 22 years of hard work. It is the original and innovative technology with independent intellectual property rights. FSN therapy is safe, non-toxic and has no side effect. Therefore, it is easy for patients to accept.

This technical standard for FSN therapy is drafted in order to facilitate clinical study and application, strengthen the standardization of FSN teaching and training and standardize the clinical operation of FSN, by which the terms and definitions, indications and contraindications, operating procedures, exceptions and the relative handling as well as precautions are standardized.

The issuing authority of this document should note that when the declaration is in line with this document, it may involve the use of patents related to disposable FSN needle and FSN inserting device.

The issuing authority of this document has no position on the authenticity, validity and scope of the patent.

The patent holder has assured the issuing authority of this document that he is willing to negotiate with any applicant on the licensing of a patent under reasonable and non-discriminatory terms and conditions. The patent holder's statement has been filed with the issuing authority of this document.

Relevant information can be obtained through the following links:

Name of patent holder: Fu Zhonghua

Address: Room 738, Building D, World Flower City, Daxing District, Beijing, China.

Please note that some of the contents of this document may involve patents. The issuing body of this document is not responsible for identifying these patents.

Standardized Manipulations of Fu's Subcutaneous Needling

1 Scope

This standard specifies the general features of Fu's Subcutaneous Needling (FSN) therapy, including terms and definitions, indications and contraindications, operation procedure, precautions, exceptions and the relative handling.

This standard is applicable to FSN therapy.

2 Normative References

This standard has no normative references.

3 Terminology and Definition

The following terms and definitions apply to this standard.

3.1

Fu's Subcutaneous Needling

Fu's Subcutaneous Needling (FSN) uses disposable FSN needle as its tool to stimulate the subcutaneous layer by doing horizontal sweeping manipulation. Needling sites are mainly selected around or near tightened muscles that cause pain or other illnesses.

3.2

Tightened Muscle (TM)

The muscles that are still in pathologically tense state while relaxed under the condition that the central nervous system functions normally.

3.3

Pre-muscular Diseases

The diseases that cause chronic ischemia and oxygen deficit, leading to pathological tension of muscle and its subsidiary structure.

3.4

Real-muscular Diseases

Caused by pathological tension of the muscle and its subsidiary structure due to chronic ischemia and oxygen deficit.

3.5

Post-muscular Diseases

A series of diseases caused by the muscles with pathological tensions that affects other organs (for example, nerve or blood vessels) which are mostly distributed in or nearby the muscles.

3.6

Needle go-forward

Pushing the needle to a proper depth after the needle is inserted into the subcutaneous layer.

3.7

Sweeping Movement

A series of parallel and left-to-right movements of the needle in the subcutaneous layer after the needle manipulation.

3.8

Reperfusion Approach

To make TMs contract vigorously within a short time and then relax in order to supply more blood to the ischemic part. It is suggested to provide equal force back by doctors when the muscles contract. RA is often used during FSN manipulation, and it can also be used separately for treatment of mild illnesses.

4 Indications and Contraindications

4.1 Indications

All indications of FSN are related to tightened muscles.

4.1.1 Pre-muscular Diseases

Ankylosing spondylitis, rheumatoid arthritis, asthma, gout, Parkinson's disease, facial paralysis, frozen shoulder and so on.

4.1.2 Real-muscular Diseases

Cervical Spondylosis, Tennis elbow, lumbar disc herniation, chronic knee pain, ankle sprain, headache, prostatitis, weak bladder (bladder leakage), hiccups, insomnia, depression, chronic cough, habitual constipation and so on.

4.1.3 Post-muscular Diseases

Dizziness, palpitation chest tightness, local numbness, local edema, breast hyperplasia, cold disease, macular degeneration, diabetic foot, avascular necrosis of the femoral head and so on.

4.2 Contraindications

4.2.1 Patients with infectious diseases, malignant diseases, or patients with acute inflammation and fever.

4.2.2 People with spontaneous bleeding or coagulopathy, which may result in nonstop bleeding after injury.

4.2.3 Skin areas with infection, ulcer, scar or tumor.

5 Operation Steps and Requirements

5.1 Determine the Needling Point

The insertion points are chosen according to the following principles.

a) In most cases, needling points are chosen nearby TMs. It can be inserted 3~5cm up, down, left, right or oblique to the TMs.

b) Needling points are better to be nearby TMs for small area and less TMs, while insertion points are better to be far away for big area and more TMs.

c) From far to near, if there are several TMs, such as chronic cervical and lumbar pain, which is usually accompanied by abnormalities of the upper limbs and lower limbs, the insertion points should be chosen from far to near, rather than the opposite.

5.2 Needle Selection and Body Position Selection

5.2.1 Needle Selection

The FSN inserting device and FSN needle should be in accordance with the regulations of national medical device production and sales supervision(Appendix A).In order to prevent needling accidents, the disposable FSN needle should be strictly inspected each time before use. If any unqualified conditions such as packaging damage are found, the needle should be eliminated.

5.2.2 Body position

Common body positions are as follows.

a) Supine position: mainly suitable for the insertion points of head, chest, abdomen and upper and lower extremities.

b) Lateral position: mainly suitable for insertion points on either side and upper and lower extremities of the body.

c) Prone position: mainly suitable for the insertion points on the head, back, hip and lower extremities. A pillow is placed under the patient's chest, the patient's hands are folded on the forehead.

d) Orthopnea position: mainly suitable for the insertion points of neck, shoulder, upper back and upper extremity, the knees and the lower extremity regions.

e) Sitting with head down position: suitable for the insertion points of the occipital and upper neck regions.

5.3 Disinfection and Needle Insertion

5.3.1 Disinfection

Sterilize the local skin: Routine skin disinfection.

The Insertion device could be used in a single way, or be sterilized the upper part with alcoholic cotton.

5.3.2 Needle Insertion

After removing the plastic protection tube, place the needle into inserting device, make sure the side with dots is facing upward and then pull the groove back to the load situation. Hold the device with middle finger at the bottom of the device, index finger on the red trigger button and thumb on the top. As shown in Fig. 1.

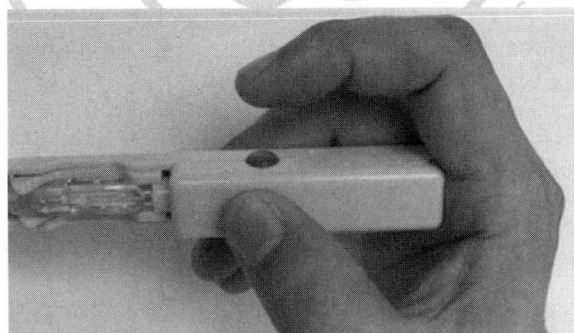

Fig.1　Gesture for holding insertion device

Place the upper part of FSN insertion device on the disinfected skin of inserting point, the angle between the device and skin should be as small as possible. With the cooperation of left hand, the operator presses the trigger button and then the needle penetrates quickly into the subcutaneous layer. As shown in Fig.2.

With left index finger and thumb holding the needle, pull the needle out of the groove, then right hand withdraws the inserting device. As shown in Fig.3

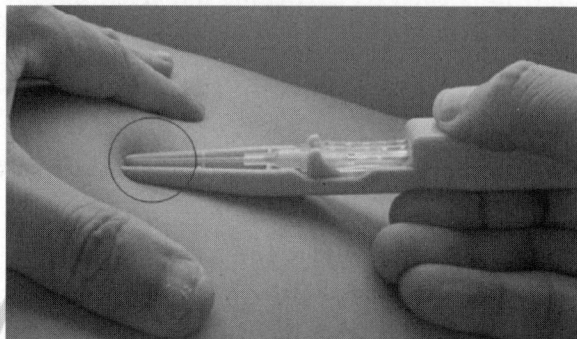

Fig. 2   Before inserting the needle, the positional relationship between inserting device and the skin

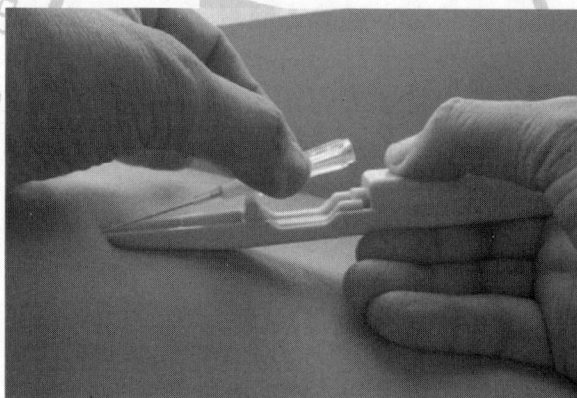

Fig. 3   After inserting, the right hand is fixed, left hand pinches the needle

5.4   Needle go-forward and Sweeping

5.4.1   Needle go-forward

After inserting the needle, if the needle is directly inserted into the muscle, the patient will feel soreness, and the practitioner's hand that is holding the needle may also feel the resistance at the same time. In this case, the practitioner should pull the needle handle with thumb, index finger and middle finger slowly backward out of the muscle layer and back to the subcutaneous layer.

After confirming the needle tip is inside the subcutaneous layer, the practitioner can put down the needle body, and then prepare for the go-forward. During which, the practitioner holds the needle with the right hand and pushes the needle forward along the subcutaneous layer. It is better to raise the needle tip slightly up when pushing, so that the tip is slightly tilted, making sure the needle does not penetrate into the muscle layer. When the needle being pushed forward, the skin is lined up. During the process, if the patient feels sudden tingling or the practitioner feels sudden resistance, it is usually because the needle tip penetrates blood vessel wall. Therefore, the needle manipulation process should be as slow as possible. When the practitioner feels the resistance before the patient feels pains, it is better to quickly withdraw the needle slightly and then adjust the needle direction upward or downward to avoid causing pains to the patient.

Generally, it is suggested to go as deep as all soft tube being under the skin. In some other cases, if the needle is inserted near the side of finger joint or other facet joints, the soft tube need not be fully embedded subcutaneously.

5.4.2 Sweeping
5.4.2.1 Sweeping Movement

When the needle is in the correct position, with the left hand fixing the soft tube seat, the practitioner can use the right hand to recede the core needle, and fix the protuberance of the soft tube seat in the slot of the core seat. At this time, the needle tip is no longer exposed outside but has returned to the soft tube, almost in line with the soft tube.

Then it is ready to perform sweeping movement. The inner nail margin of the right thumb and the middle finger are used to hold the core base, the index finger and the ring finger are separated on the left and right sides of the middle finger, and the tip of the thumb is fixed on the skin as the fulcrum. The index finger and the ring finger sweep in a seesaw-like sector one after the other. The scope of sweeping movements is better to be as large as possible, with stable speed and enough power, and sweeping rhythm should be slow so as to avoid the feeling of numbness, swelling and pain. During the sweeping process, it is suggested to use the right hand to operate while the left hand cooperates with RA.

5.4.2.2 Types of Sweeping Movement

According to different ways of swinging the needle, the sweeping movement is divided into the following two categories.

a) Horizontal sweeping movement: the sweeping action of needle tip is at the same horizontal level, which can save strength and is used more often. It can be used in most cases. Right now, with the cooperation of RA, horizontal sweeping is mostly used during clinical practice.

b) Sweeping movement in an elliptical circle: the solid needle moves clockwise or counter-clockwise under the skin to perform a circular or oval movement, applicable for intractable diseases. As Shown in Fig. 4.

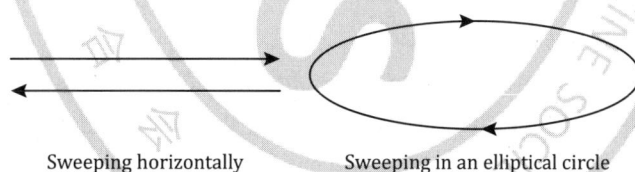

Sweeping horizontally   Sweeping in an elliptical circle

Fig. 4   Types of sweeping movement

5.4.2.3 Time and Frequency of Sweeping Movement

Each needling point can be swept for two minutes with a frequency of 200 times per minute. Practitioner can check and assess muscle tension after 30 seconds of sweeping.

5.5 Reperfusion Approach

During the FSN manipulation, reperfusion approach (RA) targeting TMs is accompanied.

5.5.1 Classification of RA

Active RA: refers to a RA that is completed by the patient without assistance.

Passive RA: refers to a RA that is completed by patients through reliance on external efforts.

5.5.2 Operational Requirements of RA

5.5.2.1 Range as Wide as Possible

According to the anatomy of the muscle and its functional activity, the practitioner should guide the patient to achieve maximum radius of the muscle (isotonic contraction) or maximum intensity of the muscle (equal length contraction).

5.5.2.2 Slow Speed

A pause of 1~3 seconds is required during the maximum radius, the maximum intensity and relaxation. It is recommended to complete a RA at around 10 seconds.

5.5.2.3 Less Number of Times

The same group of RA, which refers to activity at the same direction and the same angle, should not be repeated more than 3 times.

5.5.2.4 Length of Interval

A half-hour interval is required between two groups of reperfusion activities, so that the muscles could get enough relaxation.

5.5.2.5 Changes

Some targeted changes could be made in the RA for intractable pains.

5.5.3 Operating Methods of RA

RA is different in different parts of the body. During clinical practice, RA should be designed according to joint features and the distribution of TMs related to targeted diseases.

a) Neck: six main movements are recommended, including lowering head, raising head, turning head to the left or right side, revolving head and so on.

b) Shoulder: combing hair, trying to reach scapula of the same side, raising arms and so on.

c) Waist: holding head with hands and bowing forward on the treatment couch, flying fish posture, twisting butt from left to right, stepping movement on the same position and voluntary cough and so on.

d) Knee: flexion and extension, stepping movement on the same position.

e) Chest, back: taking deep breath, voluntary cough.

5.6 Retaining and Removing of the Soft Tube

5.6.1 Operation for Retaining the Soft Tube

When the sweeping movement is finished, the solid needle can be taken out and placed into the protective sleeve. Put a piece of adhesive tape to cover the tube seat and fix it on the skin. Make sure that the adhesive tape can cover the entire soft tube so that the soft tube kept under the skin can be fixed.

5.6.2 Time Length for Retaining the Soft Tube

It is usually suggested to retain the soft tube for 1 hour and the retaining time can vary according to different clinical situations. Doctors can decide the retaining time by taking into consideration factors like weather conditions, patient's reaction and severity of disease. If the weather is hot, the patient sweats easily or the patient has itching feeling around the needling point or surrounding area due to allergic reaction to the adhesive tape, the retaining time is better not to be long, otherwise, the retaining time can be longer.

5.6.3 Remove the Soft Tube

To remove the soft tube, use left thumb and index finger to fix surrounding skin of the needling point, then hold the soft tube seat with right thumb and index finger and take it out gently and slowly. Use a sterile cotton ball to press the needling point so as to prevent bleeding. After removal of the soft tube, patients can leave after a short break.

5.7 Time Intervals and Treatment Course

5.7.1 Time Intervals

Chronic diseases can be treated on a daily base for 2 to 3 continuous treatment, and then the time interval can be prolonged to 2 to 3 days between two treatments. For other problems, the time interval can be decided according to the treatment effect.

5.7.2 Treatment Course

Three times of treatment are usually considered as a course of treatment.

6 Exception and Its Handling

6.1 Subcutaneous Bruises

A small amount of subcutaneous bleeding and local small pieces of bruising will disappear and recover automatically, generally no special treatment is needed. But practitioners need to explain to the patient so as to eliminate the patient's worries and fears.

If the local swelling and pain is obvious or the bruised area is large and affect functional activities, practitioners need to withdraw the needle immediately and apply cold compresses to stop bleeding. After 24 hours, hot compress and mild massage can be applied to promote the dissipation of blood stasis.

6.2 Fainting during the Treatment

6.2.1 Prevention of Fainting during Treatment

It is better to explain thoroughly to the patient so as to eliminate the patient's worries, choose the right position, and treat the patient in a gentle way. If the patient feels hungry and tired, treatment can be given after the patient finishes eating, drinking and taking a rest. Supine position is recommended when patients feel too nervous. Practitioners should observe the patients' responses and ask about their feelings. If the treatment causes discomfort and the patient shows symptoms of fainting, the practitioner should stop immediately and take some necessary measures in advance.

6.2.2 Management of Fainting during Treatment

The needling operation should be stopped immediately. The practitioner should withdraw the needle, help the patients lie on bed and keep them warm. Generally, the patient will recover soon after drinking warm water or sugar water and taking some rest. If the patient is still unconscious or breathing weakly, or his or her blood pressure drops rapidly, other rescuing measures or first aid treatment should be carried out.

7 Precautions

7.1 It is suggested to give a brief explanation to patients about FSN manipulation and its features before giving treatment so as to reduce the patient's fear and doubts.

7.2 For patients who are aged and weak, the first time to receive FSN treatment and patients who are scared of needles, it is suggested to treat them by supine position.

7.3 When giving RA, the scope of activity should be from small to large, step by step, and the external force given from outside should be from light to heavy. The external force should be counterforce when patients move actively. A sudden force or vigorous activity is forbidden when giving passive activity. Age, physical, mental state and other factors of patients should be considered when practitioners design the reperfusion activities. It is better to avoid the situation that one single RA takes too much time, too much strength or is repeated too frequently.

7.4 During the period of retaining the soft tube, patients should keep adhesive tape clean and dry so as to avoid infections. Mild activities are suggested during the retaining of the soft tube but strong and large movements should be avoided in order not to affect the fixation of the soft tube. In some rare cases, if the retaining tube reaches the blood vessels, resulting in stinging or bleeding, the tube should be taken out immediately. Do not be worried if patients feel itching around the tube-retaining area, as it is usually due to allergic reactions of patients to the soft tube or adhesive tape. Practitioners can choose other kinds of materials instead to fix the tube, for example, bandages can be used.

7.5 Practitioners should not perform FSN therapy on the abdomen of women within three months of pregnancy. Even for women who are pregnant over three months, it is better not to conduct needling on the lumbosacral region and abdomen. If pregnant women are nervous, it is forbidden to do needling treatment.

7.6 If patients use safflower oil, massage milk and other stimulating drugs for external use on their skin, or receive treatment of strong plaster, strong cupping and scraping method, FSN therapy should not be applied in a short time. But if the skin condition has returned to normal after these treatments, then it is suitable to do FSN therapy.

7.7 It is better not to give FSN therapy to people who have recently received steroids injection therapy.

APPENDIX A

(Normative Appendix)

Structure and Specification of FSN

A.1   FSN Inserting Device

FSN inserting device is a device specifically designed for the inserting of FSN needle, which is developed by Nanjing FSN Medical Co. Ltd. It is convenient for therapist to deliver the needle. It can not only reduce the pain of needle insertion but also ensure the accuracy and safety of the needling. The device consists of four parts, the base, the control button, the needle drive rod and the groove, as shown in Fig. A.1.

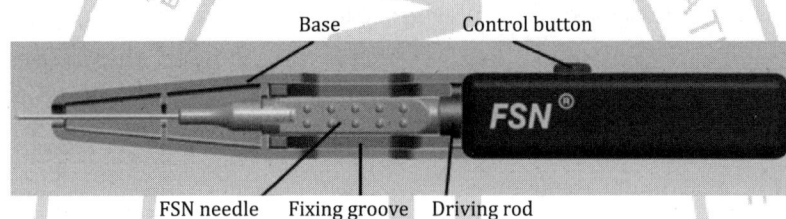

Fig. A.1   A FSN inserting device with a FSN needle

A.2   FSN Needle

A.2.1   The Structure of the FSN Needle

The FSN needle consists of three components. The combination of the three components is shown in Fig. A.2.

A.2.1.1   FSN Needle Core

The needle core consists of a stainless-steel needle and a hard-plastic core, as shown in Fig. A.2. This part insures the FSN needle to reach enough rigidity to enter the body quickly and to complete sweeping movement. The stainless-steel needle tip is bevelled. On the base, there are ten protuberances which are on one side. When the convex protuberances are upward, the bevelled tip of the needle is also upward. The surface is in line with the tip of the needle, the front end of the needle has a longitudinal groove, and the front of the groove has a transverse slot on the right side, which is used for fixing the soft casting tube during performing a sweeping movement.

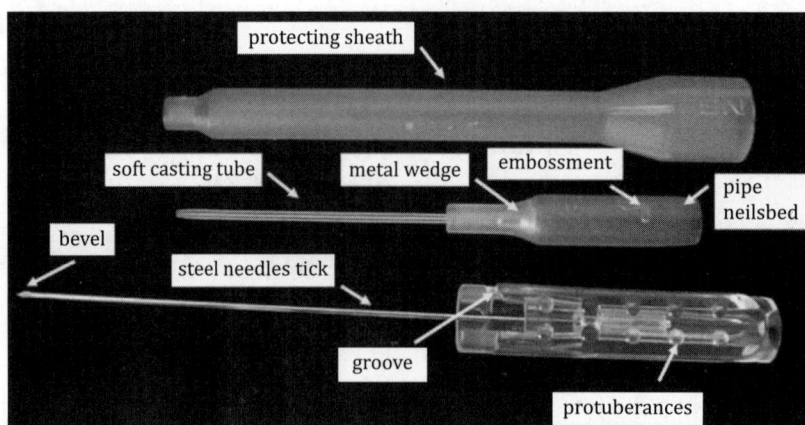

Fig. A.2   The three parts of FSN needle

A.2.1.2   Soft Casting Tube and Base of FSN Needle

The soft casting tube covers the stainless steel needle (steel needle inside, soft casting tube outside). The soft casting tube is fixed to the plastic socket through the built-in rivets, as shown in Fig. A.2. The casting tube of FSN needle has a bump, which is matched with the grooves in the core seat and the slot. The protuberances on the base are placed at the bottom of the groove when we sweep the needle.

The main function of the soft casting tube.

a) The tube and the core are anastomosed into one, which is conductive to the stability of the insertion, as well as to the needle manipulation and the sweeping movement.

b) When performing sweeping movement, the stainless steel needle tip is fully retreated into the soft tube, it can prevent the tingling caused by injuring the blood vessels.

c) Because of its sufficient softness, the tube which will not affect normal activities of patients can be kept under the skin for several hours after the treatment, and it will not puncture blood vessels and other tissues.

A2.1.3   Protective Sheath

To protect the stainless-steel needle and soft tube from the impact of the collision, we designed a protective sheath. The protective sheath is used to protect the aseptic state, as shown in Fig. A.2. After the sweeping movement, the solid needle should not be discarded. It must be put back into the protective sheath to prevent puncturing oneself and others.

A.2.2   Length, Diameter, Appearance and Preservation of FSN Needle

A.2.2.1   Appearance of FSN Needle

FSN needle is disposable and can only be used for one time, it is also known as disposable subcutaneous acupuncture needle with plastic tube, as shown in Fig. A.3 and Table A.1.

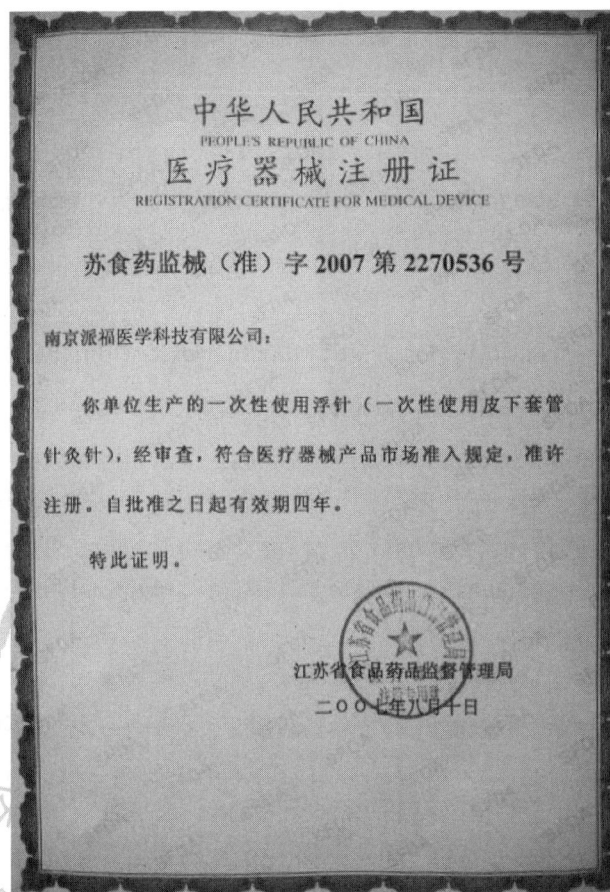

中华人民共和国
PEOPLE'S REPUBLIC OF CHINA
医疗器械注册证
REGISTRATION CERTIFICATE FOR MEDICAL DEVICE

苏食药监械（准）字 2007 第 2270536 号

南京派福医学科技有限公司：

你单位生产的一次性使用浮针（一次性使用皮下套管针灸针），经审查，符合医疗器械产品市场准入规定，准许注册。自批准之日起有效期四年。

特此证明。

江苏省食品药品监督管理局
二〇〇七年八月十日

Fig. A.3   The first Registration Certificate of FSN needle

Table A.1   The Size of the FSN Needle

	Solid Needle(mm)	Soft Tube(mm)
Length	52	49
Diameter	0.6	1.05

A.2.2.2   Use and Storage of FSN Needles

The FSN needle is a pre-sterilized product for disposable use. Please do not use once the package is damaged. After opening the package, you must make sure that the surface of the needle is bright and clean, the needle is not rough and defective, the casting tube is transparent, and the needle is sharp. If any problem is found, please stop using it and notify the manufacturer immediately.

The FSN needle should be kept in a dry, cool area.

APPENDIX B

(Data Appendix)

The Characteristics, Grading, Clinical Manifestations and Examination Methods of TMs

B.1   Basic Characteristics of Pathological Tight Muscle and its Clinical Evaluation

B.1.1   Basic Characteristics of Pathological Tight Muscle

When patients relax their inspected area and their central nervous systems function normally, doctors can still feel the "tightness, stiffness, hardness, slipperiness" feelings when touching the targeting muscles with finger pulps. Patients often have spontaneous discomfort, pains or obvious abnormal sensations. The joints that are associated with TMs are often weak and lack of strength. The range of joint activities is often reduced.

B.1.2   The Clinical Evaluation of Tightened Muscles

The muscle tension states are divided into 5 grades in clinical practice, which are defined as follows.

-: Muscles are soft and their activities are normal.

+: There is mild muscle tension without obvious clinical symptoms.

++: Muscles are moderately strained and stiff and are often accompanied by clinical symptoms which can often be relieved after a break.

+++: Muscles are tense and stiff with associated pains and other symptoms.

++++: Muscles are severely tense and stiff and if touched with finger pulps, some changes like clumps and abnormal muscular band on the muscle belly can be felt. Severe intolerable painful symptoms are often accompanied. There is no relief after a break and it even affects normal life.

B.2   Clinical Manifestations of Pathological Tight Muscles

Clinical manifestations of TMs can be divided into five major categories, including symptoms caused by TM directly or indirectly, by muscular internal organs, by dysfunctions of sleep and emotions and those with unknown reasons.

B.2.1   The First Major Category

Clinical chief complaints that are directly caused by TMs: pain, dysfunction and lack of power. The main diseases include cervical spondylosis, tennis elbow, lumbar disc herniation, chronic knee pain and ankle sprain and etc.

The characteristics of muscle-induced pains.

a) Pains that are usually characterized by sourness, swelling, or tingling in rare cases.

b) Pain positioning is often inaccurate and patients usually can only point out vague directions.

c) Peripheral muscle tissues or synergistic muscles are often affected.

d) Most of the pains can be relieved by hot compress and massage, but not by pressure. Simple touching or rubbing the skin has no effect on the pain.

e) Degree of pain may aggravate when influenced by cool weather, muscle fatigue, lack of sleep and bad mood.

f) Pain tends to decrease after using non-steroidal analgesics, after the related muscles are relaxed, the weather gets warmer, receiving massage and encountering emotional pleasure.

g) Long-term pain often causes changes in related bones and joints, such as hyperosteogeny, pseudospondylolisthesis, scoliosis, knee deformity, etc.

B.2.2 The Second Major Category

TMs affect the internal or nearby nerves, arteries and veins.

a) The main manifestations related to the affected nerves are the downstream symptoms of TMs, such as numbness.

b) The main manifestations related to the affected arteries are symptoms caused by TMs, such as headache, dizziness, chills, aversion to cold, contact temperature dropping, even cold feeling of the whole body.

c) The main manifestations related to the affected veins are the downstream symptoms caused by TMs, such as edema, heaviness, itching, and skin darkening.

B.2.3 The Third Category

Pathological tension of neighboring skeletal muscles and muscular visceral lesions affect the body at the same time and there is a close relationship between them. Both of them often appear at the same time and disappear simultaneously after treatment.

The clinical manifestations of the TMs which belong to different systems of the human body are as follows.

a) Symptoms related to smooth muscles of respiratory system include: dry cough, chronic cough, asthma, chest short breath and breathing disorders, etc.

b) Symptoms related to heart muscle include: chest tightness, palpitations, shortness of breath, chest pain, etc.

c) Symptoms related to gastrointestinal smooth muscles include: stomach bloating, heartburn, acid regurgitation, belching, loss of appetite, emaciation, habitual constipation, chronic diarrhea, afraid of cold food cold drinks, etc.

d) Symptoms related to smooth muscles of the urinary system include: urinary frequency, urgency, ureteral calculus, urine leakage, etc.

e) Symptoms related to smooth muscles of the reproductive and urinary system include.

1) Female: dysmenorrhea, menstrual abnormalities.

2) Male: impotence, etc.

B.2.4 The Fourth Category

Symptoms related to mood and sleep, anxiety, insomnia and mood swings.

B.2.5 The Fifth Category

A class of symptoms due to unknown causes, related to autonomic nervous dysfunctions and proprioceptive disorders.

Symptoms related to autonomic nervous dysfunction, such as abnormal sweating, continuous tears, continuous catarrhal rhinitis, excessive salivate, discomfort of chest areas. Symptoms related to proprioceptive disorders, such as imbalance, dizziness, tinnitus, weakness, weight perception disorders.

B.3   How to check TMs

a) Mark the patient's painful positions.

b)List all possible muscles based on anatomical and biomechanical knowledge.

c) Use thumb pulp or pulps of index finger middle finger and ring finger to touch the muscular tensions of suspected muscles. If the muscular tension of one muscle is higher than its surrounding area, it can be diagnosed as pathological tight muscle.

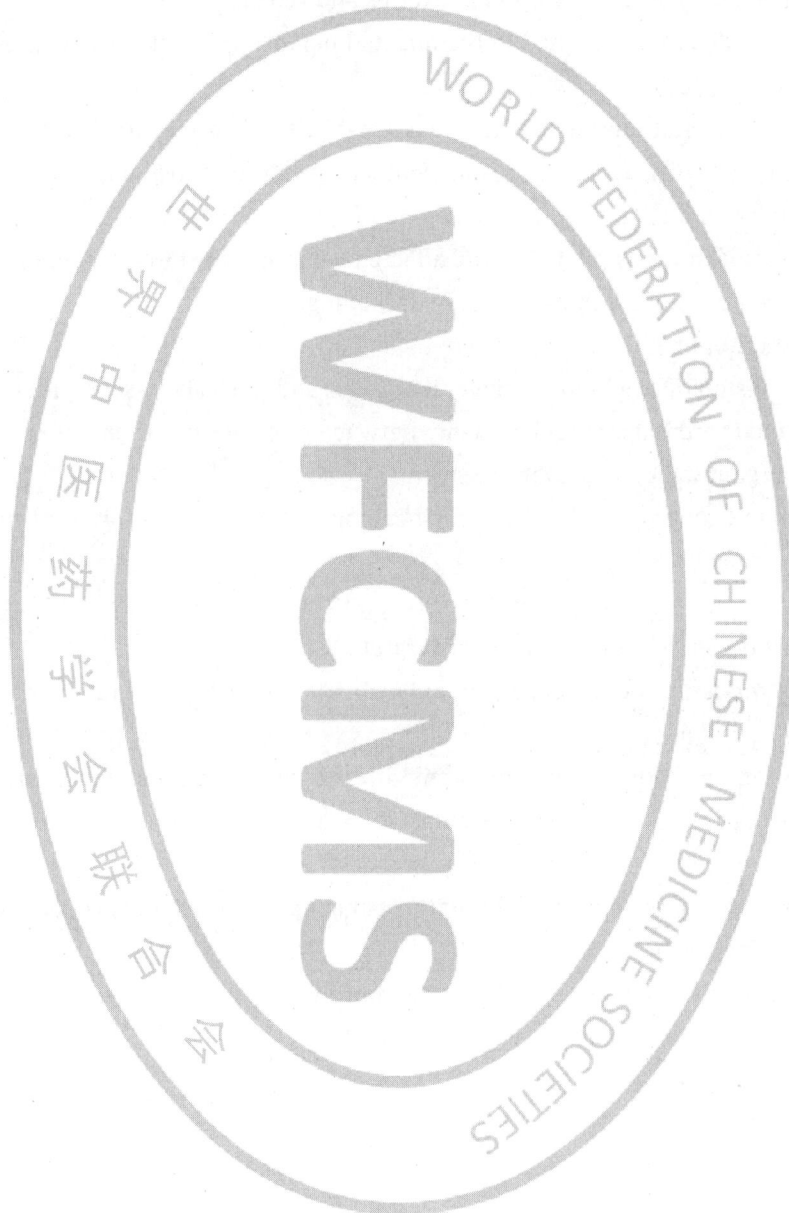

Bibliography

[1] Fu ZH. The Foundation of Fu's Subcutaneous Needling [M] . Beijing: People's Medical Publishing House, 2016.

[2] Fu ZH. The Manual of Fu's Subcutaneous Needling for Painful Problems [M] . Beijing: People's Medical Publishing House, 2011.

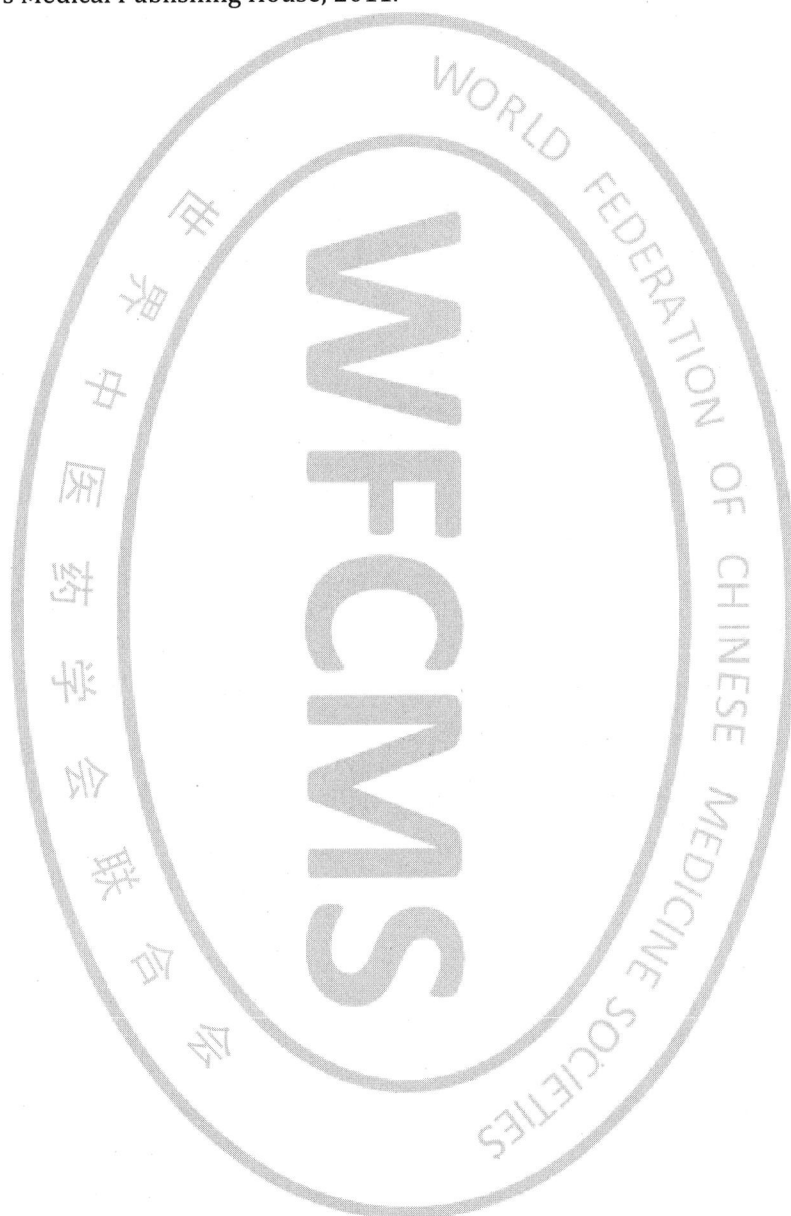